THE WINNING ENDOMETRIOSIS DIET COOKBOOK

Nourishing Low FODMAP Recipes to Alleviate Symptoms, Manage Pain, Balance Your Hormones and Reduce Body Inflammation

Steve Bryant, MD, RD

Copyright Page

Copyright © 2024 Steve Bryant, MD, RD

Table of Contents

INTRODUCTION

ello, and welcome to an exciting gastronomic journey crafted to empower and enrich individuals navigating the challenges of endometriosis. this cookbook represents a genuine commitment to provide you with delicious and nutritious meals, alongside comprehensive guidance on dietary strategies that can assist in alleviating endometriosis symptoms and enhancing your overall well-being.

endometriosis is a complex condition that affects a significant portion of the population and can profoundly impact their quality of life. it extends beyond physical health, impacting mental and social well-being as well. through the medium of culinary art, this cookbook aspires to offer comfort, education, and empowerment.

within these pages lie an array of recipes carefully crafted to meet the unique nutritional needs of individuals living with endometriosis. these dishes are not merely about satisfying hunger; they are designed to harness the healing potential of specific What You Need. from alleviating pain and fatigue to reducing inflammation, these recipes can play a vital role in your journey toward greater wellness.

yet, this cookbook transcends the role of a mere collection of dishes. it serves as a valuable resource, providing insight into the latest medical research exploring the link between endometriosis and dietary choices. delving deep into the interplay between nutrition and inflammation, hormonal balance, and digestive health, you will gain an understanding of cellular nourishment, the impact of anti-inflammatory foods, and the significance of hormone regulation.

this cookbook will empower you to incorporate nutritional strategies into your overall wellness plan as you navigate life with endometriosis. every dish, from morning meals to evening dinners, snacks to desserts, has been curated not only for its palatability but also for its contribution to the healing process.

feel no sense of isolation as you embark on this journey of exploring new cuisines and culinary techniques. countless individuals are traversing a similar path, seeking comfort and discovering the power of food. consider this cookbook as a trusted companion, equipping you with the knowledge to make delectable and healthful choices. as you strive for improved health with endometriosis, may these dishes bring you comfort, joy, and renewed vitality.

Chapter 1: What Is Endometriosis Diet Cookbook?

In the realm of dietary considerations, individuals grappling with endometriosis confront a unique set of needs and constraints, and The Endometriosis Diet Cookbook emerges as a beacon of assistance in navigating these challenges. Endometriosis, characterized by the aberrant growth of tissue akin to the uterine lining outside the uterus, often manifests in debilitating symptoms such as pain, inflammation, and discomfort. This cookbook transcends mere culinary compilation; it endeavors to illuminate the potential of specific dietary interventions in alleviating symptoms and fostering holistic well-being.

The impact of endometriosis on various facets of an individual's existence—physical comfort, mental equilibrium, and overall quality of life—is profound. Recognizing the multifaceted nature of this condition, The Endometriosis Diet Cookbook presents a holistic approach to symptom management through dietary modifications. Its array of recipes is meticulously curated in alignment with established dietary principles aimed at addressing issues ranging from inflammation to hormone regulation, thus offering a comprehensive strategy for symptom relief and improved health outcomes.

Far beyond a mere repository of recipes, this cookbook serves as an educational resource, delving into the scientific underpinnings of endometriosis and its intricate relationship with nutrition. It highlights specific foods and minerals renowned for their potential in mitigating inflammation and restoring hormonal equilibrium. The overarching objective is to empower readers with knowledge that enables informed dietary choices conducive to inflammation reduction and hormone balance maintenance.

The Endometriosis Diet Cookbook transcends its role as a mere nutritional guide; it assumes the mantle of a manual for harnessing the transformative potential of food to enhance one's health and vitality. Its repertoire spans the entirety of daily nutritional requirements, spanning from nourishing breakfast options to satisfying dinner selections, complete with tantalizing snacks and desserts. Each dish is meticulously crafted not only to deliver essential nutrients but also to evoke culinary pleasure, acknowledging the intrinsic link between food enjoyment and sustained adherence to healthy eating habits.

Through a diverse array of information and recipes, this cookbook endeavors to facilitate the enhancement of health and vitality, whether the objective is to alleviate the burden of endometriosis-related symptoms or to pursue optimal well-being more broadly. It stands as a testament to the remarkable healing capacity of food and extends a helping hand to individuals striving to embrace a fuller, more joyous existence in spite of the challenges posed by endometriosis.

Significance of Adhering to the Endometriosis Dietary Plan

The Endometriosis Diet holds profound significance as it stands poised to offer relief to individuals grappling with the debilitating symptoms of endometriosis, enabling them to reclaim control over their lives and enhance their overall quality of life. Endometriosis, characterized by the abnormal growth of uterine-like tissue in unexpected locations within the body, often leads to chronic pain, inflammation, and a myriad of other distressing symptoms that profoundly impact daily functioning and well-being. In response to these challenges, the Endometriosis Diet emerges as a specialized dietary approach aimed at alleviating pain symptoms and fostering improved health outcomes.

Central to the Endometriosis Diet is its focus on combatting chronic inflammation, a key contributor to the development and exacerbation of endometriosis-related symptoms. By emphasizing the consumption of anti-inflammatory foods rich in antioxidants, omega-3 fatty acids, and similar compounds, this dietary approach seeks to mitigate inflammation levels within the body, thereby offering potential relief from pain and discomfort.

Moreover, the Endometriosis Diet recognizes the pivotal role of hormonal balance in managing endometriosis symptoms effectively. Given that endometriosis is profoundly influenced by hormonal fluctuations, dietary interventions targeting hormonal equilibrium become paramount. By incorporating foods known to support hormonal homeostasis and alleviate symptoms associated with hormonal imbalances, such as those experienced during premenstrual syndrome (PMS), individuals may experience enhanced symptom management and overall well-being.

Furthermore, the Endometriosis Diet places a strong emphasis on nurturing gastrointestinal health, reflecting emerging research highlighting the intricate interplay between gut health and endometriosis. Through the inclusion of prebiotic and probiotic-rich foods, this dietary approach seeks to cultivate a favorable gut microbiota, which in turn may bolster immune function and attenuate inflammation, offering potential benefits for individuals with endometriosis.

Beyond symptom alleviation, the Endometriosis Diet empowers individuals to take an active role in their health and well-being through informed dietary choices. By fostering a sense of agency and control over one's body and health outcomes, this dietary approach instills confidence and optimism, fostering a renewed sense of vitality and zest for life.

The Endometriosis Diet acknowledges that navigating the complexities of endometriosis is a deeply personal journey. Serving as a flexible framework for understanding the role of nutrition in symptom management and health promotion, this dietary approach offers individuals the tools and resources needed to tailor their dietary practices to their unique needs and preferences. By embracing the principles outlined in the Endometriosis Diet, individuals may embark on a path towards improved health, reduced pain, and enhanced overall well-being, thereby reclaiming agency over their lives amidst the challenges

posed by endometriosis.

Chapter 2: Managing Endometriosis through Diet

Endometriosis sufferers possess the agency to adopt a proactive and multifaceted approach to managing their condition by integrating strategic dietary modifications into their daily routines. Endometriosis, characterized by the abnormal growth of tissue resembling the uterine lining outside the uterus, often manifests with chronic pain, inflammation, and a myriad of distressing symptoms. Recognizing the intricate interplay among nutrition, inflammation, hormone balance, and gut health is pivotal in shaping a dietary regimen tailored to address the unique needs and challenges associated with endometriosis.

A key aspect of the endometriosis diet revolves around mitigating inflammation, which significantly contributes to the development and exacerbation of symptoms associated with the condition. Dietary choices play a pivotal role in modulating inflammation levels within the body. Incorporating anti-inflammatory foods such as fatty fish, flaxseeds, and walnuts, alongside antioxidant-rich fruits and vegetables, holds promise in alleviating pain and reducing inflammation levels.

Furthermore, restoring hormonal equilibrium emerges as a central tenet of the endometriosis diet, as hormonal fluctuations exert a profound influence on the presence and intensity of symptoms experienced. Hormonal imbalances can trigger discomfort, bloating, and mood fluctuations, yet selecting meals that support hormonal balance offers potential relief. Foods abundant in fiber, healthy fats, and cruciferous vegetables like broccoli and kale are instrumental in promoting hormonal health and mitigating symptom severity.

Additionally, mounting evidence underscores the pivotal role of gut health in the management of endometriosis. Recent research highlights a plausible link between intestinal health and the severity of the condition, underscoring the importance of dietary interventions that foster a thriving microbiome within the digestive tract. Prioritizing prebiotic foods such as garlic, onions, and asparagus, alongside probiotic-rich options like yogurt and fermented foods, fosters a favorable gut environment, thereby bolstering immune function and mitigating inflammation.

Integral to the endometriosis diet is the conscientious avoidance of dietary triggers that exacerbate inflammation and disrupt hormonal balance. Limiting or abstaining from the consumption of processed foods, refined sugars, and excessive amounts of coffee and alcohol can create a conducive environment for symptom management and overall well-being.

It is essential to acknowledge that there is no one-size-fits-all solution when it comes to the endometriosis diet, as individual responses to the condition vary widely. Thus, seeking personalized guidance from healthcare professionals or registered dietitians specializing in endometriosis is imperative to ensure that dietary choices align with individual health needs and goals.

Incorporating strategic dietary modifications into the management of endometriosis represents a comprehensive and proactive strategy aimed at empowering individuals to take control of their health and reduce symptom burden. By prioritizing foods that are anti-inflammatory, hormone-balancing, and gut-nourishing while minimizing dietary irritants, individuals with endometriosis can enhance their quality of life and regain a sense of agency over their health journey. The endometriosis diet serves as a powerful tool for self-empowerment, enabling individuals to make informed decisions that support their well-being and foster a sense of vitality and resilience.

The fundamental tenets of the Endometriosis Diet

The concept of the Endometriosis Diet embodies a comprehensive and personalized approach to dietary management aimed at enhancing the well-being of individuals grappling with endometriosis. By targeting symptom reduction, inflammation mitigation, and overall health improvement, this dietary framework offers a nuanced roadmap for informed and health-enhancing dietary choices, taking into account the intricate interplay between nutrition, inflammation, hormone equilibrium, and gut health.

Central to the Endometriosis Diet is its emphasis on anti-inflammatory strategies as a means to alleviate symptoms associated with the condition. Recognizing that discomfort and suffering in endometriosis often stem from inflammation, the diet incorporates a plethora of anti-inflammatory components. Examples include antioxidants and omega-3 fatty acids found abundantly in colorful fruits and vegetables, fatty fish, nuts, seeds, and olive oil. By embracing such dietary choices, individuals may experience a reduction in inflammation and the amelioration of associated symptoms.

Moreover, the Endometriosis Diet recognizes the significance of adequate nutrient intake in restoring hormonal balance, a crucial factor in managing symptoms effectively. Foods rich in fiber, healthy fats, vitamins, and minerals take precedence in promoting hormonal equilibrium. Incorporating a variety of whole grains, lean meats, cruciferous vegetables, and omega-3 fatty acid sources into the diet can aid in maintaining hormonal balance and alleviating symptom severity.

Recent research has unveiled a compelling link between gut health and the severity of endometriosis symptoms, prompting a proactive approach to nurturing a healthy gut microbiota within the Endometriosis Diet. Prebiotic-rich foods such as garlic, onions, and artichokes support the proliferation of beneficial gut bacteria, while probiotic-rich options like yogurt and fermented foods foster microbial diversity. By prioritizing gut health, individuals may witness improvements in immune function, inflammation modulation, and overall symptom management.

Conversely, the Endometriosis Diet advises against foods that may exacerbate inflammation and hormonal imbalances, thereby worsening symptoms. Processed foods, refined carbohydrates, caffeine, and alcohol are singled out as potential triggers to be limited or eliminated from the diet. By reducing exposure to these inflammatory agents, individuals may experience a reduction in symptom severity and overall improvement in health outcomes.

Recognizing the unique nature of each individual's experience with endometriosis, the Endometriosis Diet underscores the importance of customization and personalization in dietary management. Acknowledging that a one-size-fits-all approach may not suffice, the diet encourages individuals to monitor their responses to different foods, maintain food diaries if necessary, and tailor their dietary choices accordingly. Seeking guidance from healthcare professionals or registered dietitians specializing in endometriosis is recommended to ensure personalized and effective dietary strategies.

Nutrients for Maintaining Hormonal Equilibrium

For individuals grappling with the challenges of endometriosis, hormonal imbalances can exacerbate symptoms and significantly impact overall well-being. In navigating this complex landscape, the role of nutrients emerges as paramount in promoting hormonal equilibrium and alleviating discomfort. The Endometriosis Diet underscores the significance of specific nutrients in fostering hormonal balance, pain relief, and holistic wellness.

Omega-3 fatty acids, abundant in foods such as salmon, mackerel, sardines, flaxseeds, walnuts, and other fatty fish, stand out as potent allies in combating inflammation and mitigating the discomfort associated with endometriosis. These beneficial fats not only possess anti-inflammatory properties but also offer potential relief from symptoms, underscoring their therapeutic value.

Furthermore, a diet rich in fiber from whole grains, legumes, vegetables, and fruits emerges as instrumental in supporting hormonal harmony.

By stabilizing blood sugar levels and facilitating proper digestion, fiber contributes to mitigating hormonal fluctuations and promoting overall well-being. Additionally, fiber aids in the excretion of unwanted hormones, further enhancing its role in hormonal regulation.

Vitamin D assumes a crucial role in maintaining hormonal and immune system health, with optimal levels contributing to reduced inflammation and alleviation of endometriosis-related pain. Sun exposure and dietary sources such as fatty fish, fortified dairy products, and egg yolks serve as avenues for bolstering vitamin D levels and supporting symptom management.

B vitamins, including B6, B12, and folate, exert profound effects on mood regulation, hormone synthesis, and cellular metabolism. B6, in particular, plays a pivotal role in neurotransmitter and hormone production, while vitamin B12 and folate are essential for proper cell metabolism and overall hormonal balance.

Zinc, a vital mineral, plays a pivotal role in hormone synthesis, particularly those crucial for reproduction. Adequate zinc intake not only helps prevent endometriosis symptoms but also supports regular menstrual cycles, highlighting its significance in hormonal health.

Magnesium emerges as a multifaceted nutrient with implications for restful sleep, mood regulation, and hormonal balance. Abundant in nuts, seeds, whole grains, and dark leafy greens, magnesium aids in minimizing muscle stress and discomfort associated with endometriosis, thereby contributing to overall well-being.

Selenium, an antioxidant mineral, holds promise in mitigating inflammation and maintaining balanced hormone levels. Foods rich in selenium, such as Brazil nuts, seafood, and whole grains, offer valuable support in managing endometriosis symptoms and promoting hormonal equilibrium.

Furthermore, iron supplementation is imperative for endometriosis patients to prevent anemia resulting from excessive menstrual bleeding. Incorporating iron-rich foods such as lean meats, beans, lentils, and dark leafy greens into the diet helps maintain energy levels and overall health.

Chapter 3: Supplements for Endometriosis

Introducing supplements into an endometriosis management regimen can serve as a valuable adjunct therapy, potentially alleviating symptoms and enhancing overall health. Certain vitamins and nutrients have demonstrated promise in addressing various aspects of endometriosis; however, it is imperative to seek guidance from a healthcare professional before initiating any supplement regimen, ensuring safety and appropriateness.

Omega-3 fatty acids, obtained from sources such as fish oil or algae, offer potent anti-inflammatory properties that can help mitigate the inflammation associated with endometriosis. Incorporating these supplements into one's routine may provide relief from discomfort and support inflammatory management.

Many individuals with endometriosis exhibit low levels of vitamin D, a nutrient essential for immune function and inflammation regulation. Supplementing with vitamin D can help maintain optimal levels, potentially aiding in inflammation management and symptom alleviation. Prior to supplementation, it is advisable to undergo testing to determine existing vitamin D levels.

Supplementation with magnesium has been shown to alleviate muscular tension and promote relaxation. The muscle-relaxing properties of magnesium can be particularly beneficial in easing the pain and spasms commonly experienced by individuals with endometriosis.

Curcumin, the active compound in turmeric, boasts potent anti-inflammatory effects that may help reduce inflammation and alleviate endometriosis-related pain. Enhancing curcumin's bioavailability through co-administration with black pepper or specialized supplements can optimize its effectiveness.

Iron supplements may prove beneficial for individuals experiencing heavy menstrual bleeding associated with endometriosis, helping to mitigate fatigue and other symptoms of anemia. Coordination with dietary adjustments, as advised by a healthcare provider, is recommended when incorporating iron supplementation.

Vitamins B6 and B12 play pivotal roles in hormone regulation and overall well-being. A comprehensive vitamin B complex supplement can provide a spectrum of B vitamins necessary for energy production, mood regulation, and hormone metabolism.

Given the potential link between gut microbiota health and inflammation, probiotics may offer promise in managing endometriosis symptoms. Supplementation with probiotics can foster a healthy gut microbiome, potentially bolstering immunity and attenuating inflammation.

Dietary supplements such as turmeric and pine bark extract (Pycnogenol) have garnered attention for their potential to alleviate pain and inflammation associated with endometriosis. Monitoring individual responses is essential, as outcomes may vary.

Evening primrose oil capsules are reported to provide relief for some individuals with endometriosis, particularly in alleviating sore breasts and discomfort. However, individual responses can vary, underscoring the importance of careful observation and tracking.

Prior consultation with a healthcare provider is paramount before initiating any new supplement regimen, as certain supplements may entail risks or interact with prescribed medications. Additionally, attention to supplement quality and dosage is crucial when making selections.

While supplements may offer support in managing endometriosis symptoms, they are not a substitute for a well-rounded, nutrient-rich diet. A holistic approach encompassing dietary modifications, lifestyle adjustments, and medical oversight remains the cornerstone of comprehensive endometriosis management, ensuring optimal symptom control and overall well-being.

Alleviating Symptoms of Endometriosis

For individuals grappling with the challenges posed by endometriosis, alleviating symptoms stands as a paramount objective. Fortunately, a plethora of strategies exist to aid in achieving this goal, each offering a unique avenue towards symptom management. Endometriosis, characterized by its hallmark symptoms of pain, inflammation, and various discomforts, arises from the presence of tissue akin to the uterine lining proliferating outside the confines of the uterus. While no singular panacea exists, a multifaceted approach encompassing diverse interventions holds promise in ameliorating symptomatology.

Among the arsenal of interventions, the Endometriosis Diet emerges as a noteworthy contender, emphasizing dietary choices that harbor anti-inflammatory properties, foster hormonal equilibrium, and nurture gut health. Incorporating a rich array of fruits, vegetables, whole grains, lean proteins, and healthy fats into one's diet can effectively mitigate inflammation and stabilize hormone levels. Concurrently, minimizing the consumption of coffee, alcohol, refined carbohydrates, and processed foods may contribute to symptom alleviation.

Furthermore, supplementation, under the guidance of healthcare professionals, offers targeted support in managing endometriosis symptoms. Omega-3 fatty acids, vitamin D, magnesium, and curcumin represent examples of supplements that have demonstrated efficacy in attenuating inflammation and discomfort associated with endometriosis. However, it is imperative to seek medical advice before initiating any supplementation regimen to ensure appropriateness and safety.

Over-the-counter nonsteroidal anti-inflammatory drugs (NSAIDs) such as ibuprofen serve as accessible options for pain management, albeit with caution regarding prolonged usage, necessitating consultation with a healthcare provider. Similarly, heat therapy, in the form of heating pads, can provide relief by relaxing pelvic muscles and alleviating discomfort.

Moreover, engaging in regular exercise and physical activity yields multifaceted benefits for individuals with endometriosis, facilitating pain reduction through enhanced blood circulation and endorphin release. Activities such as yoga and gentle stretching hold promise in symptom management by promoting relaxation and mobility.

Stress management practices, encompassing meditation, deep breathing exercises, mindfulness techniques, and relaxation activities, offer avenues for reducing stress-related inflammation and fostering tranquility.

Prioritizing good sleep hygiene emerges as a fundamental aspect of symptom management, as adequate rest supports discomfort reduction and overall health enhancement. Establishing a consistent sleep schedule, creating a conducive sleep environment, and incorporating relaxation rituals before bedtime contribute to optimizing sleep quality.

A balanced diet, coupled with hydration, forms the cornerstone of a healthy lifestyle conducive to managing endometriosis symptoms. Adequate nutrition provides essential nutrients for hormonal balance and immune function, while hydration aids in digestion and inflammation modulation.

Chapter 4: Inflammation-Fighting Dishes

RECOMMENDED BREAKFAST RECIPES

Quinoa Porridge with Berries and Almond Milk:

What You Need

1/2 cup quinoa

1 cup almond milk

1 cup mixed berries (such as strawberries, blueberries, raspberries)

How To Make

Rinse quinoa under cold water and drain.

In a saucepan, combine quinoa and almond milk. Bring to a boil, then reduce heat to a simmer.

Cover and cook for about 15 minutes or until quinoa is tender and the liquid is absorbed.

Serve in a bowl and top with mixed berries.

Scrambled Tofu with Spinach and Tomatoes:

What You Need

1/2 block of firm tofu, crumbled

1 cup fresh spinach leaves

1/2 cup cherry tomatoes, halved

1 tablespoon olive oil

1/2 teaspoon turmeric

Salt and pepper to taste

How To Make

Heat olive oil in a skillet over medium heat.

Add crumbled tofu and sauté for 2-3 minutes.

Sprinkle turmeric, salt, and pepper over the tofu and mix well.

Add spinach and cherry tomatoes, cook for another 2 minutes until spinach wilts and tomatoes soften.

Serve hot.

Buckwheat Pancakes Topped with Greek Yogurt and Fresh Fruit:

What You Need

1 cup buckwheat flour

1 tablespoon baking powder

1 tablespoon maple syrup or honey

1 cup almond milk

1 large egg (or flaxseed egg for a vegan option)

Greek yogurt

Mixed fresh fruit (such as berries, sliced peaches, or kiwi)

How To Make

In a large bowl, whisk together buckwheat flour, baking powder, maple syrup or honey, almond milk, and egg until smooth.

Heat a non-stick pan over medium heat and lightly grease with oil.

Pour 1/4 cup of batter onto the pan for each pancake. Cook until bubbles form on the surface, then flip and cook until golden brown on both sides.

Serve pancakes topped with a dollop of Greek yogurt and mixed fresh fruit.

Smoothie with Kale, Banana, Blueberries, and Almond Milk:

What You Need

1 cup kale leaves, stems removed

1 ripe banana

1/2 cup blueberries

1 cup almond milk

1 tablespoon almond butter (optional)

Ice cubes (optional)

How To Make

In a blender, add kale, banana, blueberries, almond milk, and almond butter (if using).

Blend until smooth and creamy. If desired, add ice cubes and blend again for a cold smoothie.

Pour into a glass and enjoy.

Avocado Toast with Poached Eggs and Hemp Seeds:

What You Need

2 slices whole-grain bread

1 ripe avocado

2 poached eggs

Hemp seeds

Salt and pepper to taste

How To Make

Toast the whole-grain bread slices.

Mash the ripe avocado and spread it evenly on the toasted bread.

Top each slice with a poached egg.

Sprinkle hemp seeds, salt, and pepper over the eggs.

Serve immediately.

Chia Seed Pudding with Sliced Fruits and Honey:

What You Need

1/4 cup chia seeds

1 cup almond milk

1 tablespoon honey

Sliced fruits (such as mango, kiwi, or banana)

How To Make

In a bowl, mix chia seeds and almond milk. Stir well to avoid clumps.

Let the mixture sit for at least 2 hours or overnight in the refrigerator until it thickens.

Add honey and stir to combine.

Serve in a glass and top with sliced fruits.

Brown Rice Cakes with Avocado and Smoked Salmon:

What You Need

2 brown rice cakes

1 ripe avocado

Smoked salmon slices

Lemon juice

Fresh dill or chives (optional)

Salt and pepper to taste

How To Make

Slice the avocado and mash it lightly with a fork. Drizzle lemon juice over the avocado and season with salt and pepper.

Spread the avocado mixture on the brown rice cakes.

Top with smoked salmon slices.

Garnish with fresh dill or chives if desired.

Serve as an open-faced sandwich.

Overnight Oats with Grated Carrot, Raisins, and Coconut Flakes:

What You Need

1/2 cup rolled oats

1 cup almond milk

1/2 cup grated carrot

1/4 cup raisins

1 tablespoon honey or maple syrup

1 tablespoon coconut flakes

How To Make

In a jar or container, combine rolled oats, almond milk, grated carrot, raisins, and honey or maple syrup.

Stir well to mix all the What You Need.

Cover the jar or container and refrigerate overnight.

In the morning, give it a stir and top with coconut flakes before serving.

Veggie Omelet with Mushrooms, Spinach, and Bell Peppers:

What You Need

3 large eggs

1/4 cup sliced mushrooms

1 cup fresh spinach leaves

1/4 cup sliced bell peppers (any color)

1 tablespoon olive oil

Salt and pepper to taste

How To Make

In a bowl, whisk the eggs with a pinch of salt and pepper.

Heat olive oil in a non-stick skillet over medium heat.

Add mushrooms and bell peppers, sauté for 2-3 minutes until they soften.

Add spinach and cook for another minute until wilted.

Pour the whisked eggs into the skillet, tilting the pan to spread them evenly.

Cook until the omelet is set and slightly browned on the bottom, then fold it in half.

Slide the omelet onto a plate and serve.

Almond Butter and Banana Sandwich on Whole-Grain Bread:

What You Need

2 slices whole-grain bread

2 tablespoons almond butter

1 ripe banana, thinly sliced

How To Make

Spread almond butter on one slice of bread.

Place banana slices on top of the almond
butter.

Top with the other slice of bread to make a
sandwich.

Press gently to hold everything together.

Cut the sandwich in half if desired and enjoy.

Spinach and Mushroom Frittata with a Side of Mixed Greens:

What You Need

4 large eggs

1 cup fresh spinach leaves

1/2 cup sliced mushrooms

1/4 cup diced onions

1 tablespoon olive oil

Salt and pepper to taste

Mixed greens for serving

How To Make

Preheat the oven to 375°F (190°C).

In a bowl, whisk the eggs with salt and pepper.

Heat olive oil in an oven-safe skillet over medium heat.

Add onions and mushrooms, sauté until onions are translucent and mushrooms are cooked.

Add spinach and cook until wilted.

Pour the whisked eggs over the vegetables in the skillet, making sure they are evenly distributed.

Cook on the stovetop for 1-2 minutes until the edges start to set.

Transfer the skillet to the preheated oven and bake for about 10 minutes or until the frittata is cooked through and lightly browned on top.

Slice the frittata into wedges and serve with a side of mixed greens.

Oatmeal with Flaxseeds, Nuts, and Cinnamon:

What You Need

1/2 cup rolled oats

1 cup water or almond milk

1 tablespoon ground flaxseeds

2 tablespoons chopped nuts (such as almonds or walnuts)

1/2 teaspoon ground cinnamon

How To Make

In a saucepan, bring water or almond milk to a boil.

Stir in the rolled oats and reduce heat to low. Cook for about 5 minutes or until the oats are creamy.

Remove from heat and stir in ground flaxseeds, chopped nuts, and ground cinnamon.

Serve in a bowl.

Greek Yogurt Parfait with Granola and Mixed Berries:

What You Need

1 cup Greek yogurt

1/4 cup granola (choose a low-sugar option)

1/2 cup mixed berries (such as strawberries, blueberries, raspberries)

How To Make

In a glass or bowl, layer Greek yogurt, granola, and mixed berries.

Repeat the layers until all What You Need are used.

You can add a drizzle of honey or maple syrup for added sweetness if desired.

Serve the parfait immediately or refrigerate for later.

Quinoa Breakfast Bowl with Roasted Vegetables and Tahini Dressing:

What You Need

1/2 cup cooked quinoa

Assorted roasted vegetables (such as sweet potatoes, zucchini, and cherry tomatoes)

1 tablespoon tahini

1 tablespoon lemon juice

1 tablespoon water

Salt and pepper to taste

Fresh herbs for garnish (such as parsley or cilantro)

How To Make

In a bowl, assemble the cooked quinoa and roasted vegetables.

In a small bowl, whisk together tahini, lemon juice, water, salt, and pepper to make the dressing.

Drizzle the tahini dressing over the quinoa and vegetables.

Garnish with fresh herbs and serve.

Sweet Potato Hash with Black Beans and Avocado Slices:

What You Need

1 large sweet potato, peeled and diced

1/2 cup cooked black beans

1/2 avocado, sliced

1 tablespoon olive oil

1/2 teaspoon ground cumin

1/4 teaspoon chili powder

Salt and pepper to taste

How To Make

In a skillet, heat olive oil over medium heat.

Add diced sweet potato and sauté until tender and slightly crispy.

Stir in cooked black beans, ground cumin, chili powder, salt, and pepper.

Cook for another 2 minutes to combine the flavors.

Serve the sweet potato hash with sliced avocado on top.

RECOMMENDED LUNCH RECIPES

Quinoa Salad with Roasted Vegetables and Lemon-Tahini Dressing:

What You Need

1 cup cooked quinoa

Assorted roasted vegetables (such as bell peppers, zucchini, and cherry tomatoes)

2 tablespoons tahini

1 tablespoon lemon juice

1 tablespoon water

Salt and pepper to taste

Fresh herbs for garnish (such as parsley or cilantro)

How To Make

In a bowl, assemble the cooked quinoa and roasted vegetables.

In a small bowl, whisk together tahini, lemon juice, water, salt, and pepper to make the dressing.

Drizzle the lemon-tahini dressing over the quinoa and vegetables.

Garnish with fresh herbs and serve.

Zucchini Noodles with Pesto Sauce and Cherry Tomatoes:

What You Need

2 large zucchini, spiralized or cut into thin noodles

Pesto sauce (store-bought or homemade)

Cherry tomatoes, halved

Fresh basil leaves for garnish

How To Make

In a skillet, sauté zucchini noodles over medium heat for 2-3 minutes until slightly softened.

Toss the zucchini noodles with pesto sauce until they are evenly coated.

Add halved cherry tomatoes to the skillet and cook for another minute.

Garnish with fresh basil leaves and serve.

Grilled Chicken or Tofu Wraps with Hummus and Veggies:

What You Need

Grilled chicken breast or tofu slices

Whole-grain tortillas or wraps

Hummus

Sliced cucumbers

Sliced tomatoes

Baby spinach leaves

How To Make

Lay the whole-grain tortillas or wraps flat.

Spread a layer of hummus on each wrap.

Add grilled chicken or tofu slices, sliced cucumbers, sliced tomatoes, and baby spinach leaves on top.

Roll the wraps tightly and cut in half if desired.

Turkey or Tempeh Lettuce Wraps with Cucumber and Carrot Slaw:

What You Need

Ground turkey or crumbled tempeh

Lettuce leaves (such as iceberg or butter lettuce)

Shredded cucumber and carrot slaw (use a julienne peeler or grater)

Hoisin sauce or peanut sauce (store-bought or homemade)

Chopped green onions and cilantro for garnish

How To Make

In a skillet, cook ground turkey or tempeh over medium heat until fully cooked and seasoned with desired spices (if using turkey).

Lay out lettuce leaves and spoon the cooked turkey or tempeh onto each leaf.

Top with shredded cucumber and carrot slaw.

Drizzle hoisin sauce or peanut sauce over the wraps.

Garnish with chopped green onions and cilantro.

Baked Sweet Potato topped with Black Beans, Salsa, and Guacamole:

What You Need

2 medium sweet potatoes

1 can black beans, drained and rinsed

Salsa (store-bought or homemade)

Guacamole (store-bought or homemade)

Fresh cilantro for garnish

How To Make

Preheat the oven to 400°F (200°C).

Wash the sweet potatoes and pierce them with a fork.

Place the sweet potatoes on a baking sheet and bake for 40-50 minutes until tender.

Slice each sweet potato open and fluff the flesh with a fork.

Top each sweet potato with black beans, salsa, and guacamole.

Garnish with fresh cilantro and serve.

Spinach and Feta Stuffed Bell Peppers with a Side of Quinoa:

What You Need

2 large bell peppers (any color)

1 cup cooked quinoa

1 cup fresh spinach leaves

1/2 cup crumbled feta cheese

1 tablespoon olive oil

1/2 teaspoon dried oregano

Salt and pepper to taste

How To Make

Preheat the oven to 375°F (190°C).

Cut the tops off the bell peppers and remove the seeds and membranes.

In a skillet, heat olive oil over medium heat.

Add fresh spinach leaves and sauté until wilted.

In a bowl, mix cooked quinoa, sautéed spinach, crumbled feta cheese, dried oregano, salt, and pepper.

Stuff each bell pepper with the quinoa mixture.

Place the stuffed bell peppers on a baking dish and bake in the preheated oven for about 20-25 minutes or until the peppers are tender.

Lentil and Vegetable Soup with a Side of Mixed Greens:

What You Need

1 cup cooked lentils (green or brown)

Assorted chopped vegetables (such as carrots, celery, and onions)

4 cups vegetable broth

1 tablespoon olive oil

1 teaspoon dried thyme

Salt and pepper to taste

Mixed greens for serving

How To Make

In a pot, heat olive oil over medium heat.

Add chopped vegetables and sauté until they start to soften.

Add cooked lentils, vegetable broth, dried thyme, salt, and pepper.

Bring to a boil, then reduce heat and simmer for about 15-20 minutes.

Serve the lentil and vegetable soup with a side of mixed greens.

Cauliflower Rice Stir-Fry with Shrimp or Tofu:

What You Need

1 small head of cauliflower, riced (using a food processor or grater)

1 cup cooked shrimp or cubed tofu

Assorted chopped vegetables (such as broccoli, bell peppers, and snap peas)

2 tablespoons soy sauce (or tamari for gluten-free option)

1 tablespoon sesame oil

1 tablespoon rice vinegar

1 teaspoon minced ginger

2 garlic cloves, minced

Green onions and sesame seeds for garnish

How To Make

In a wok or large skillet, heat sesame oil over medium-high heat.

Add minced ginger and garlic, sauté for 1 minute until fragrant.

Add chopped vegetables and stir-fry until they are crisp-tender.

Stir in cauliflower rice and cooked shrimp or tofu.

Pour soy sauce and rice vinegar over the stir-fry and toss to combine.

Garnish with chopped green onions and sesame seeds.

Brown Rice Bowl with Baked Salmon, Avocado, and Steamed Broccoli:

What You Need

1 cup cooked brown rice

Baked salmon fillet (seasoned with lemon, dill, and salt)

1 ripe avocado, sliced

Steamed broccoli florets

Lemon wedges for serving

How To Make

In a bowl, assemble the cooked brown rice, baked salmon, sliced avocado, and steamed broccoli.

Squeeze lemon juice over the bowl for extra flavor if desired.

Serve the brown rice bowl with a side of lemon wedges.

Mediterranean Chickpea Salad with Cucumber, Tomato, and Olives:

What You Need

1 can chickpeas, drained and rinsed

1 large cucumber, diced

1 cup cherry tomatoes, halved

1/2 cup pitted Kalamata olives

1/4 cup diced red onion

2 tablespoons extra-virgin olive oil

1 tablespoon lemon juice

1 teaspoon dried oregano

Salt and pepper to taste

Crumbled feta cheese (optional)

Fresh parsley for garnish

How To Make

In a large bowl, combine chickpeas, diced cucumber, cherry tomatoes, olives, and red onion.

In a small bowl, whisk together extra-virgin olive oil, lemon juice, dried oregano, salt, and pepper to make the dressing.

Pour the dressing over the salad and toss to coat all the What You Need.

If desired, sprinkle crumbled feta cheese on top.

Garnish with fresh parsley and serve.

Baked Cod with Lemon and Herbs, served with Steamed Asparagus:

What You Need

Cod fillets

Lemon slices

Fresh herbs (such as thyme or dill)

Salt and pepper to taste

Fresh asparagus spears

How To Make

Preheat the oven to 375°F (190°C).

Season the cod fillets with salt, pepper, and fresh herbs.

Place the cod fillets on a baking sheet lined with parchment paper.

Top each fillet with lemon slices.

Bake in the preheated oven for about 12-15 minutes or until the cod is cooked through and flaky.

While the cod is baking, steam the asparagus spears until tender-crisp.

Serve the baked cod with a side of steamed asparagus.

Grilled Vegetable Sandwich on Whole-Grain Bread:

What You Need

Assorted grilled vegetables (such as eggplant, zucchini, and bell peppers)

Whole-grain bread slices

Hummus or pesto sauce (store-bought or homemade)

Fresh baby spinach or arugula leaves

How To Make

Lay the whole-grain bread slices flat.

Spread a layer of hummus or pesto sauce on each slice.

Add grilled vegetables and fresh baby spinach or arugula leaves on one slice.

Top with the other slice of bread to make a sandwich.

Press gently to hold everything together.

Cut the sandwich in half if desired and enjoy.

Spinach and Mushroom Frittata with a Side of Mixed Greens:

What You Need

4 large eggs

1 cup fresh spinach leaves

1/2 cup sliced mushrooms

1/4 cup diced onions

1 tablespoon olive oil

Salt and pepper to taste

Mixed greens for serving

How To Make

Preheat the oven to 375°F (190°C).

In a bowl, whisk the eggs with a pinch of salt and pepper.

Heat olive oil in an oven-safe skillet over medium heat.

Add diced onions and sliced mushrooms, sauté until onions are translucent and mushrooms are cooked.

Add fresh spinach and cook until wilted.

Pour the whisked eggs into the skillet, tilting the pan to spread them evenly.

Cook on the stovetop for 1-2 minutes until the edges start to set.

Transfer the skillet to the preheated oven and bake for about 10 minutes or until the frittata is cooked through and lightly browned on top.

Slice the frittata into wedges and serve with a side of mixed greens.

Quinoa Bowl with Roasted Butternut Squash, Kale, and Goat Cheese:

What You Need

1 cup cooked quinoa

Roasted butternut squash cubes

Sautéed kale (with garlic and olive oil)

Crumbled goat cheese

Toasted pumpkin seeds or chopped pecans for garnish (optional)

How To Make

In a bowl, assemble the cooked quinoa, roasted butternut squash, and sautéed kale.

Top with crumbled goat cheese.

If desired, sprinkle toasted pumpkin seeds or chopped pecans on top for added texture and flavor.

Chickpea and Vegetable Stir-Fry with Quinoa:

What You Need

1 cup cooked quinoa

1 can chickpeas, drained and rinsed

Assorted chopped vegetables (such as bell peppers, snap peas, and carrots)

2 tablespoons soy sauce (or tamari for gluten-free option)

1 tablespoon sesame oil

1 tablespoon rice vinegar

1 teaspoon minced ginger

1 garlic clove, minced

Sesame seeds for garnish (optional)

How To Make

In a wok or large skillet, heat sesame oil over medium-high heat.

Add minced ginger and garlic, sauté for 1 minute until fragrant.

Add chopped vegetables and stir-fry until they are crisp-tender.

Stir in cooked quinoa and chickpeas.

Pour soy sauce and rice vinegar over the stir-fry and toss to combine.

Garnish with sesame seeds if desired and serve.

RECOMMENDED DINNER RECIPES

Baked Salmon with Quinoa and Roasted Vegetables:

What You Need

2 salmon fillets

1 cup quinoa

Assorted roasted vegetables (such as broccoli, carrots, and bell peppers)

Olive oil

Lemon wedges

Fresh dill or parsley for garnish

Salt and pepper to taste

How To Make

Preheat the oven to 375°F (190°C).

Place the salmon fillets on a baking sheet lined with parchment paper.

Drizzle olive oil over the salmon and season with salt and pepper.

Bake in the preheated oven for about 12-15 minutes or until the salmon is cooked through and flakes easily with a fork.

While the salmon is baking, cook the quinoa according to package How To Make.

Roast the vegetables in the oven with a little olive oil until tender.

Serve the baked salmon on a bed of quinoa and roasted vegetables.

Garnish with lemon wedges, fresh dill, or parsley.

Stuffed Bell Peppers with Quinoa and Black Beans:

What You Need

4 large bell peppers (any color)

1 cup cooked quinoa

1 can black beans, drained and rinsed

1 cup diced tomatoes (canned or fresh)

1 cup chopped spinach

1/2 cup diced onions

2 cloves garlic, minced

1 tablespoon olive oil

1 teaspoon ground cumin

Salt and pepper to taste

Shredded cheese (optional)

How To Make

Preheat the oven to 375°F (190°C).

Cut the tops off the bell peppers and remove the seeds and membranes.

In a skillet, heat olive oil over medium heat.

Add diced onions and minced garlic, sauté until onions are translucent.

Stir in chopped spinach, ground cumin, salt, and pepper.

Add cooked quinoa, black beans, and diced tomatoes to the skillet. Mix well to combine.

Stuff each bell pepper with the quinoa and black bean mixture.

Place the stuffed bell peppers on a baking dish and bake in the preheated oven for about 25-30 minutes or until the peppers are tender.

If desired, sprinkle shredded cheese on top of the stuffed peppers during the last 5 minutes of baking.

Zucchini Noodles with Tomato Sauce and Turkey Meatballs:

What You Need

4 medium zucchini, spiralized or cut into thin noodles

1 jar tomato sauce (store-bought or homemade)

Turkey meatballs (store-bought or homemade)

Fresh basil leaves for garnish

Shaved Parmesan cheese (optional)

How To Make

In a large skillet, warm the tomato sauce over medium heat.

Add turkey meatballs to the sauce and simmer until heated through.

While the meatballs are simmering, sauté the zucchini noodles in a separate pan until tender.

Serve the zucchini noodles topped with tomato sauce and turkey meatballs.

Garnish with fresh basil leaves and shaved Parmesan cheese if desired.

Baked Cod with Lemon and Herbs, served with Asparagus and Quinoa:

What You Need

Cod fillets

Lemon slices

Fresh herbs (such as thyme or dill)

Salt and pepper to taste

Fresh asparagus spears

1 cup quinoa

Olive oil

How To Make

Preheat the oven to 375°F (190°C).

Season the cod fillets with salt, pepper, and fresh herbs.

Place the cod fillets on a baking sheet lined with parchment paper.

Top each fillet with lemon slices.

Bake in the preheated oven for about 12-15 minutes or until the cod is cooked through and flakes easily with a fork.

While the cod is baking, cook the quinoa according to package How To Make.

Steam the asparagus spears until tender-crisp.

Serve the baked cod with a side of steamed asparagus and quinoa.

Lentil Curry with Cauliflower Rice:

What You Need

1 cup dried red lentils

1 small head of cauliflower, riced (using a food processor or grater)

1 can coconut milk

2 tablespoons curry powder

1 tablespoon olive oil

1 onion, diced

2 cloves garlic, minced

1-inch piece of ginger, minced

1 can diced tomatoes

Salt and pepper to taste

Fresh cilantro for garnish

How To Make

In a large pot, heat olive oil over medium heat.

Add diced onions, minced garlic, and minced ginger. Sauté until the onions are translucent.

Stir in curry powder and cook for another minute until fragrant.

Add red lentils, coconut milk, and diced tomatoes to the pot. Bring to a boil, then reduce heat and simmer for about 15-20 minutes until the lentils are tender and the curry thickens.

While the lentil curry is simmering, prepare the cauliflower rice by ricing the cauliflower using a food processor or grater.

Season the cauliflower rice with salt and pepper and steam it until tender.

Serve the lentil curry over a bed of cauliflower rice and garnish with fresh cilantro.

Chickpea and Vegetable Tagine with Couscous:

What You Need

1 can chickpeas, drained and rinsed

Assorted chopped vegetables (such as carrots, sweet potatoes, and bell peppers)

1 onion, diced

2 cloves garlic, minced

1-inch piece of ginger, minced

1 can diced tomatoes

2 cups vegetable broth

1 tablespoon olive oil

1 teaspoon ground cumin

1 teaspoon ground coriander

1 teaspoon ground cinnamon

Salt and pepper to taste

Fresh cilantro for garnish

Cooked couscous

How To Make

In a large pot or tagine, heat olive oil over medium heat.

Add diced onions, minced garlic, and minced ginger. Sauté until the onions are translucent.

Stir in ground cumin, ground coriander, ground cinnamon, salt, and pepper.

Add chopped vegetables, chickpeas, diced tomatoes, and vegetable broth to the pot. Bring to a boil, then reduce heat and simmer for about 20-25 minutes until the vegetables are tender and the flavors meld.

Serve the chickpea and vegetable tagine over cooked couscous.

Garnish with fresh cilantro.

Butternut Squash and Spinach Risotto:

What You Need

1 cup Arborio rice (risotto rice)

4 cups vegetable broth

2 cups diced butternut squash

2 cups fresh spinach leaves

1/2 cup diced onions

2 cloves garlic, minced

2 tablespoons olive oil

1/4 cup grated Parmesan cheese (optional for garnish)

Salt and pepper to taste

Fresh sage leaves for garnish

How To Make

In a large pot, heat olive oil over medium heat.

Add diced onions and minced garlic, sauté until onions are translucent.

Stir in Arborio rice and cook for 1-2 minutes until lightly toasted.

Add diced butternut squash and a ladleful of vegetable broth to the pot. Stir frequently and allow the rice to absorb the broth.

Continue adding the vegetable broth, one ladleful at a time, stirring frequently, until the rice is creamy and cooked al dente (about 20-25 minutes).

Stir in fresh spinach leaves until wilted.

Season the risotto with salt and pepper to taste.

Serve the butternut squash and spinach risotto with grated Parmesan cheese (optional) and garnish with fresh sage leaves.

Quinoa and Vegetable Stir-Fry with Tofu or Tempeh:

What You Need

1 cup cooked quinoa

Assorted chopped vegetables (such as broccoli, carrots, and snap peas)

1 block tofu or tempeh, cubed

2 tablespoons soy sauce (or tamari for gluten-free option)

1 tablespoon sesame oil

1 tablespoon rice vinegar

1 teaspoon minced ginger

2 garlic cloves, minced

Sesame seeds for garnish (optional)

How To Make

In a wok or large skillet, heat sesame oil over medium-high heat.

Add minced ginger and garlic, sauté for 1 minute until fragrant.

Add chopped vegetables and stir-fry until they are crisp-tender.

Add cubed tofu or tempeh and cook until heated through.

Pour soy sauce and rice vinegar over the stir-fry and toss to combine.

Serve the quinoa and vegetable stir-fry with a sprinkle of sesame seeds if desired.

Turkey or Lentil Lettuce Wraps with Cucumber and Carrot Slaw:

What You Need

Ground turkey or cooked lentils

Lettuce leaves (such as iceberg or butter lettuce)

Shredded cucumber and carrot slaw (use a julienne peeler or grater)

Hoisin sauce or peanut sauce (store-bought or homemade)

Chopped green onions and cilantro for garnish

How To Make

In a skillet, cook ground turkey until fully cooked and seasoned with desired spices (if using turkey) or heat up cooked lentils.

Lay out lettuce leaves and spoon the cooked turkey or lentils onto each leaf.

Top with shredded cucumber and carrot slaw.

Drizzle hoisin sauce or peanut sauce over the wraps.

Garnish with chopped green onions and cilantro.

Grilled Chicken or Tofu with Steamed Broccoli and Sweet Potato:

What You Need

Chicken breasts or tofu slices

2 sweet potatoes, peeled and cubed

2 cups broccoli florets

Olive oil

Salt and pepper to taste

How To Make

Preheat the grill or grill pan over medium-high heat.

Drizzle olive oil over the chicken breasts or tofu slices and season with salt and pepper.

Grill the chicken or tofu for about 4-5 minutes per side or until fully cooked and nicely charred.

While grilling the protein, steam the sweet potato cubes until tender.

Steam the broccoli until crisp-tender.

Serve the grilled chicken or tofu with a side of steamed broccoli and sweet potato cubes.

Grilled Portobello Mushrooms with a Side of Mixed Greens:

What You Need

4 large Portobello mushrooms

2 tablespoons balsamic vinegar

2 tablespoons olive oil

2 cloves garlic, minced

Salt and pepper to taste

Mixed greens salad (with your choice of dressing)

How To Make

Preheat the grill or grill pan over medium-high heat.

In a small bowl, whisk together balsamic vinegar, olive oil, minced garlic, salt, and pepper.

Brush the Portobello mushrooms with the balsamic mixture on both sides.

Grill the mushrooms for about 5-6 minutes per side or until tender and grill marks appear.

Serve the grilled Portobello mushrooms with a side of mixed greens salad.

Eggplant Parmesan with a Side of Arugula Salad:

What You Need

1 large eggplant, sliced into rounds

1 cup breadcrumbs (use gluten-free breadcrumbs if needed)

2 eggs (or flaxseed mixture for a vegan option)

1 jar marinara sauce (store-bought or homemade)

Shredded mozzarella cheese (use dairy-free cheese for a vegan option)

Fresh basil leaves for garnish

Arugula salad (with your choice of dressing)

How To Make

Preheat the oven to 375°F (190°C).

Dip eggplant slices in beaten eggs or flaxseed mixture, then coat them with breadcrumbs.

Place the breaded eggplant slices on a baking sheet lined with parchment paper.

Bake in the preheated oven for about 15-20 minutes or until the eggplant is tender and crispy.

In a separate baking dish, layer marinara sauce, baked eggplant slices, and shredded mozzarella cheese.

Repeat the layers until all What You Need are used, finishing with a layer of cheese on top.

Bake the Eggplant Parmesan in the oven for another 10-15 minutes or until the cheese is melted and bubbly.

Garnish with fresh basil leaves.

Serve the Eggplant Parmesan with a side of arugula salad.

Black Bean and Sweet Potato Tacos with Avocado Cream:

What You Need

1 can black beans, drained and rinsed

2 large sweet potatoes, peeled and cubed

1 tablespoon olive oil

1 teaspoon ground cumin

1 teaspoon chili powder

Salt and pepper to taste

Corn or flour tortillas (choose gluten-free tortillas if needed)

Avocado cream (blend avocado, lime juice, garlic, salt, and pepper until smooth)

Fresh cilantro for garnish

How To Make

Preheat the oven to 400°F (200°C).

Toss the cubed sweet potatoes with olive oil, ground cumin, chili powder, salt, and pepper.

Spread the sweet potatoes on a baking sheet lined with parchment paper.

Roast in the preheated oven for about 20-25 minutes or until the sweet potatoes are tender and lightly browned.

In a separate pan, heat the black beans until warmed through.

Warm the tortillas in a dry skillet or directly over a gas flame until pliable.

Assemble the tacos with a layer of black beans, roasted sweet potatoes, and a dollop of avocado cream.

Garnish with fresh cilantro.

Stuffed Acorn Squash with Wild Rice and Cranberries:

What You Need

2 acorn squashes, halved and seeds removed

1 cup wild rice

2 cups vegetable broth

1/2 cup dried cranberries

1/4 cup chopped pecans or walnuts (optional)

1 tablespoon olive oil

1 tablespoon maple syrup

Salt and pepper to taste

Fresh parsley for garnish

How To Make

Preheat the oven to 375°F (190°C).

Place the acorn squash halves on a baking sheet lined with parchment paper.

Drizzle olive oil and maple syrup over the squash halves, then season with salt and pepper.

Roast the acorn squash in the preheated oven for about 35-40 minutes or until tender.

While the squash is roasting, cook the wild rice in vegetable broth according to package How To Make.

Stir in dried cranberries and chopped pecans or walnuts into the cooked wild rice.

Once the squash is tender, fill each halve with the wild rice and cranberry mixture.

Garnish with fresh parsley.

RECOMMENDED RECOMMENDED SOUP RECIPES

Spinach and Chickpea Soup:

What You Need

1 can chickpeas, drained and rinsed

4 cups vegetable broth

1 tablespoon olive oil

1 onion, diced

2 cloves garlic, minced

1 teaspoon ground cumin

1/2 teaspoon ground coriander

4 cups fresh spinach leaves

Salt and pepper to taste

Lemon wedges for garnish

How To Make

In a large pot, heat olive oil over medium heat.

Add diced onions and sauté until they become translucent.

Stir in minced garlic and cook for another minute until fragrant.

Add ground cumin, ground coriander, chickpeas, and vegetable broth to the pot.

Bring the mixture to a boil, then reduce heat and simmer for about 10-15 minutes.

Stir in fresh spinach leaves and cook until wilted.

Season the soup with salt and pepper to taste.

Serve the Spinach and Chickpea soup hot, garnished with lemon wedges.

Carrot Ginger Soup:

What You Need

1 pound carrots, peeled and chopped

1 tablespoon olive oil

1 onion, diced

2 cloves garlic, minced

1-inch piece of ginger, peeled and minced

4 cups vegetable broth

1 cup coconut milk (or almond milk for a lighter option)

Salt and pepper to taste

Fresh cilantro for garnish

How To Make

In a large pot, heat olive oil over medium heat.

Add diced onions and sauté until they become translucent.

Stir in minced garlic and ginger, and cook for another minute until fragrant.

Add chopped carrots and vegetable broth to the pot.

Bring the mixture to a boil, then reduce heat and simmer for about 20-25 minutes or until the carrots are tender.

Use an immersion blender or a regular blender to puree the soup until smooth.

Stir in coconut milk (or almond milk) to achieve the desired consistency.

Season the soup with salt and pepper to taste.

Serve the Carrot Ginger soup hot, garnished with fresh cilantro.

Creamy Broccoli Soup:

What You Need

2 cups chopped broccoli florets

1 tablespoon olive oil

1 onion, diced

2 cloves garlic, minced

4 cups vegetable broth

1 cup coconut milk (or almond milk for a lighter option)

Salt and pepper to taste

Sliced almonds for garnish (optional)

How To Make

In a large pot, heat olive oil over medium heat.

Add diced onions and sauté until they become translucent.

Stir in minced garlic and cook for another minute until fragrant.

Add chopped broccoli and vegetable broth to the pot.

Bring the mixture to a boil, then reduce heat and simmer for about 10-15 minutes or until the broccoli is tender.

Use an immersion blender or a regular blender to puree the soup until smooth.

Stir in coconut milk (or almond milk) to achieve the desired creaminess.

Season the soup with salt and pepper to taste.

Serve the Creamy Broccoli soup hot, garnished with sliced almonds if desired.

Butternut Squash Soup:

What You Need

1 medium butternut squash, peeled, seeded, and diced

1 tablespoon olive oil

1 onion, diced

2 cloves garlic, minced

4 cups vegetable broth

1/2 teaspoon ground cinnamon

1/4 teaspoon ground nutmeg

Salt and pepper to taste

Coconut milk (optional, for added creaminess)

Roasted pumpkin seeds for garnish

How To Make

In a large pot, heat olive oil over medium heat.

Add diced onions and sauté until they become translucent.

Stir in minced garlic and cook for another minute until fragrant.

Add diced butternut squash and vegetable broth to the pot.

Bring the mixture to a boil, then reduce heat and simmer for about 20-25 minutes or until the squash is tender.

Use an immersion blender or a regular blender to puree the soup until smooth.

Stir in ground cinnamon, ground nutmeg, salt, and pepper.

If desired, add coconut milk for added creaminess and stir to combine.

Serve the butternut squash soup hot, garnished with roasted pumpkin seeds.

Shrimp and Vegetable Stir-Fry with Brown Rice:

What You Need

1 pound large shrimp, peeled and deveined

Assorted chopped vegetables (such as bell peppers, snap peas, and carrots)

2 tablespoons soy sauce (or tamari for gluten-free option)

1 tablespoon sesame oil

1 tablespoon rice vinegar

1 teaspoon minced ginger

2 garlic cloves, minced

Cooked brown rice

How To Make

In a wok or large skillet, heat sesame oil over medium-high heat.

Add minced ginger and garlic, sauté for 1 minute until fragrant.

Add chopped vegetables and stir-fry until they are crisp-tender.

Add shrimp and cook until they turn pink and are fully cooked.

Pour soy sauce and rice vinegar over the stir-fry and toss to combine.

Serve the shrimp and vegetable stir-fry over cooked brown rice.

Sweet Potato and Black Bean Soup:

What You Need

2 large sweet potatoes, peeled and cubed

1 tablespoon olive oil

1 onion, diced

2 cloves garlic, minced

1 can black beans, drained and rinsed

4 cups vegetable broth

1 teaspoon ground cumin

1/2 teaspoon smoked paprika

Salt and pepper to taste

Fresh cilantro for garnish

How To Make

In a large pot, heat olive oil over medium heat.

Add diced onions and sauté until they become translucent.

Stir in minced garlic and cook for another minute until fragrant.

Add cubed sweet potatoes, black beans, vegetable broth, ground cumin, and smoked paprika to the pot.

Bring the mixture to a boil, then reduce heat and simmer for about 20-25 minutes or until the sweet potatoes are tender.

Use an immersion blender or a regular blender to partially puree the soup, leaving some chunks of sweet potatoes and black beans for texture.

Season the soup with salt and pepper to taste.

Serve the Sweet Potato and Black Bean soup hot, garnished with fresh cilantro.

Curried Cauliflower Soup:

What You Need

1 large cauliflower head, chopped into florets

1 tablespoon olive oil

1 onion, diced

2 cloves garlic, minced

1 tablespoon curry powder

1 teaspoon ground turmeric

4 cups vegetable broth

1 cup coconut milk (or almond milk for a lighter option)

Salt and pepper to taste

Fresh cilantro for garnish

How To Make

Preheat the oven to 400°F (200°C).

Toss the cauliflower florets with olive oil and spread them on a baking sheet lined with parchment paper.

Roast the cauliflower in the preheated oven for about 20-25 minutes or until they are tender and lightly browned.

In a large pot, heat olive oil over medium heat.

Add diced onions and sauté until they become translucent.

Stir in minced garlic and cook for another minute until fragrant.

Add roasted cauliflower, curry powder, ground turmeric, and vegetable broth to the pot.

Bring the mixture to a boil, then reduce heat and simmer for about 10 minutes.

Use an immersion blender or a regular blender to puree the soup until smooth.

Stir in coconut milk (or almond milk) to achieve the desired creaminess.

Season the soup with salt and pepper to taste.

Serve the Curried Cauliflower soup hot, garnished with fresh cilantro.

Red Lentil and Coconut Soup:

What You Need

1 cup red lentils

4 cups vegetable broth

1 tablespoon olive oil

1 onion, diced

2 cloves garlic, minced

1 can diced tomatoes

1 can coconut milk

1 teaspoon ground cumin

1/2 teaspoon ground coriander

1/4 teaspoon cayenne pepper (optional, for heat)

Salt and pepper to taste

Fresh cilantro for garnish

How To Make

Rinse the red lentils under cold water and drain.

In a large pot, heat olive oil over medium heat.

Add diced onions and sauté until they become translucent.

Stir in minced garlic and cook for another minute until fragrant.

Add red lentils, vegetable broth, diced tomatoes, coconut milk, ground cumin, ground coriander, and cayenne pepper (if using) to the pot.

Bring the mixture to a boil, then reduce heat and simmer for about 15-20 minutes or until the lentils are tender.

Season the soup with salt and pepper to taste.

Serve the Red Lentil and Coconut soup hot, garnished with fresh cilantro.

Minestrone Soup with Whole Grain Pasta:

What You Need

1 cup whole grain pasta (such as penne or farfalle)

4 cups vegetable broth

1 tablespoon olive oil

1 onion, diced

2 carrots, diced

2 celery stalks, diced

2 cloves garlic, minced

1 can diced tomatoes

1 can kidney beans, drained and rinsed

1 teaspoon dried basil

1 teaspoon dried oregano

Salt and pepper to taste

Fresh basil leaves for garnish

How To Make

Cook the whole grain pasta according to package How To Make, then drain and set aside.

In a large pot, heat olive oil over medium heat.

Add diced onions, carrots, and celery. Sauté until the vegetables are softened.

Add minced garlic and cook for another minute until fragrant.

Stir in diced tomatoes, kidney beans, vegetable broth, dried basil, and dried oregano.

Bring the mixture to a boil, then reduce heat and simmer for about 10-15 minutes.

Season the soup with salt and pepper to taste.

Add the cooked whole grain pasta to the soup and stir to combine.

Serve the Minestrone soup hot, garnished with fresh basil leaves.

Vegetable Lentil Soup:

What You Need

1 cup dried brown or green lentils

4 cups vegetable broth

1 tablespoon olive oil

1 onion, diced

2 carrots, diced

2 celery stalks, diced

2 cloves garlic, minced

1 can diced tomatoes

1 teaspoon dried thyme

1 teaspoon dried oregano

Salt and pepper to taste

Fresh parsley for garnish

How To Make

Rinse the lentils under cold water and drain.

In a large pot, heat olive oil over medium heat.

Add diced onions, carrots, and celery. Sauté until the vegetables are softened.

Add minced garlic and cook for another minute until fragrant.

Stir in lentils, vegetable broth, diced tomatoes, dried thyme, and dried oregano.

Bring the mixture to a boil, then reduce heat and simmer for about 20-25 minutes or until the lentils are tender.

Season the soup with salt and pepper to taste.

Garnish with fresh parsley before serving.

Mushroom Barley Soup:

What You Need

1 cup pearl barley

4 cups vegetable broth

1 tablespoon olive oil

1 onion, diced

2 cloves garlic, minced

8 ounces cremini mushrooms, sliced

1 carrot, diced

1 celery stalk, diced

1 teaspoon dried thyme

1 bay leaf

Salt and pepper to taste

Fresh parsley for garnish

How To Make

Rinse the pearl barley under cold water and drain.

In a large pot, heat olive oil over medium heat.

Add diced onions, carrots, and celery. Sauté until the vegetables are softened.

Stir in minced garlic and cook for another minute until fragrant.

Add sliced cremini mushrooms, pearl barley, vegetable broth, dried thyme, and bay leaf to the pot.

Bring the mixture to a boil, then reduce heat and simmer for about 25-30 minutes or until the barley is tender.

Season the soup with salt and pepper to taste.

Remove the bay leaf before serving.

Serve the Mushroom Barley soup hot, garnished with fresh parsley.

Thai Coconut Curry Soup with Tofu:

What You Need

1 tablespoon coconut oil

1 onion, diced

2 cloves garlic, minced

1-inch piece of ginger, peeled and minced

1 tablespoon red curry paste

4 cups vegetable broth

1 can coconut milk

8 ounces firm tofu, cubed

1 red bell pepper, sliced

1 zucchini, sliced

1 tablespoon soy sauce (or tamari for gluten-free option)

Juice of 1 lime

Fresh cilantro for garnish

How To Make

In a large pot, heat coconut oil over medium heat.

Add diced onions, minced garlic, and minced ginger. Sauté until the onions are translucent.

Stir in red curry paste and cook for another minute until fragrant.

Add vegetable broth and coconut milk to the pot, and bring the mixture to a boil.

Add cubed tofu, sliced red bell pepper, and sliced zucchini.

Simmer the soup for about 10-15 minutes or until the vegetables are tender.

Stir in soy sauce and lime juice.

Season the soup with additional soy sauce or lime juice if desired.

Serve the Thai Coconut Curry soup hot, garnished with fresh cilantro.

Tomato Basil Soup with Quinoa:

What You Need

1 cup quinoa

4 cups vegetable broth

1 tablespoon olive oil

1 onion, diced

2 cloves garlic, minced

1 can diced tomatoes

2 tablespoons tomato paste

1 teaspoon dried basil

1/2 teaspoon dried thyme

Salt and pepper to taste

Fresh basil leaves for garnish

How To Make

Rinse the quinoa under cold water and drain.

In a large pot, heat olive oil over medium heat.

Add diced onions and sauté until they become translucent.

Stir in minced garlic and cook for another minute until fragrant.

Add quinoa, vegetable broth, diced tomatoes, tomato paste, dried basil, and dried thyme to the pot.

Bring the mixture to a boil, then reduce heat and simmer for about 15-20 minutes or until the quinoa is cooked and the flavors meld.

Season the soup with salt and pepper to taste.

Serve the Tomato Basil soup hot, garnished with fresh basil leaves.

Roasted Vegetable and White Bean Soup:

What You Need

2 cups chopped mixed vegetables (such as carrots, bell peppers, and squash)

1 tablespoon olive oil

1 onion, diced

2 cloves garlic, minced

1 can white beans, drained and rinsed

4 cups vegetable broth

1 teaspoon dried thyme

1 teaspoon dried rosemary

Salt and pepper to taste

Fresh parsley for garnish

How To Make

Preheat the oven to 400°F (200°C).

Toss the chopped mixed vegetables with olive oil and spread them on a baking sheet lined with parchment paper.

Roast the vegetables in the preheated oven for about 20-25 minutes or until they are tender and lightly browned.

In a large pot, heat olive oil over medium heat.

Add diced onions and sauté until they become translucent.

Stir in minced garlic and cook for another minute until fragrant.

Add roasted vegetables, white beans, vegetable broth, dried thyme, and dried rosemary to the pot.

Bring the mixture to a boil, then reduce heat and simmer for about 10 minutes.

Season the soup with salt and pepper to taste.

Serve the Roasted Vegetable and White Bean soup hot, garnished with fresh parsley.

Cabbage and White Bean Soup:

What You Need

1 tablespoon olive oil

1 onion, diced

2 cloves garlic, minced

4 cups shredded cabbage

1 can white beans, drained and rinsed

1 can diced tomatoes

4 cups vegetable broth

1 teaspoon dried thyme

1 bay leaf

Salt and pepper to taste

Fresh parsley for garnish

How To Make

In a large pot, heat olive oil over medium heat.

Add diced onions and sauté until they become translucent.

Stir in minced garlic and cook for another minute until fragrant.

Add shredded cabbage, white beans, diced tomatoes, vegetable broth, dried thyme, and bay leaf to the pot.

Bring the mixture to a boil, then reduce heat and simmer for about 15-20 minutes or until the cabbage is tender.

Season the soup with salt and pepper to taste.

Remove the bay leaf before serving.

Serve the Cabbage and White Bean soup hot, garnished with fresh parsley.

Lemon Chicken Soup with Orzo:

What You Need

1 tablespoon olive oil

1 onion, diced

2 cloves garlic, minced

4 cups chicken broth

2 boneless, skinless chicken breasts, cooked and shredded

1/2 cup uncooked orzo pasta

Juice of 1 lemon

2 tablespoons chopped fresh dill

Salt and pepper to taste

Lemon slices for garnish

How To Make

In a large pot, heat olive oil over medium heat.

Add diced onions and sauté until they become translucent.

Stir in minced garlic and cook for another minute until fragrant.

Add chicken broth and bring the mixture to a boil.

Stir in shredded cooked chicken and orzo pasta.

Simmer the soup for about 10-12 minutes or until the orzo is cooked.

Stir in lemon juice and chopped fresh dill.

Season the soup with salt and pepper to taste.

Serve the Lemon Chicken soup hot, garnished with lemon slices.

Potato Leek Soup:

What You Need

2 tablespoons butter or olive oil

2 leeks, cleaned and thinly sliced

4 cups vegetable broth

4 cups diced potatoes

1 cup milk or non-dairy milk

Salt and pepper to taste

Fresh chives for garnish

How To Make

In a large pot, melt butter or heat olive oil over medium heat.

Add sliced leeks and sauté until they become tender and slightly caramelized.

Stir in vegetable broth and diced potatoes.

Bring the mixture to a boil, then reduce heat and simmer for about 20-25 minutes or until the potatoes are soft.

Use an immersion blender or a regular blender to puree the soup until smooth.

Stir in milk (or non-dairy milk) to achieve the desired creaminess.

Season the soup with salt and pepper to taste.

Serve the Potato Leek soup hot, garnished with
fresh chives.

RECOMMENDED DESSERT RECIPES

Greek Yogurt Parfait with Fresh Berries and Honey:

What You Need

1 cup plain Greek yogurt

1 tablespoon honey

1 cup fresh mixed berries (such as strawberries, blueberries, and blackberries)

1/4 cup granola (use gluten-free granola if needed)

How To Make

In a glass or bowl, layer plain Greek yogurt, fresh mixed berries, and granola.

Drizzle honey on top of the parfait for added sweetness.

Repeat the layers to create a beautiful presentation.

Serve the Greek Yogurt Parfait with Fresh Berries and Honey as a delightful and nutritious dessert.

Banana Oatmeal Cookies:

What You Need

2 ripe bananas, mashed

1 cup rolled oats (use gluten-free oats if needed)

1/4 cup almond flour or any other flour of choice

1/4 cup unsweetened applesauce

1 teaspoon vanilla extract

1/4 cup dark chocolate chips (or dairy-free chocolate chips for a vegan option)

1/4 cup chopped walnuts or pecans (optional)

Pinch of cinnamon (optional)

How To Make

Preheat the oven to 350°F (175°C) and line a baking sheet with parchment paper.

In a mixing bowl, combine mashed bananas, rolled oats, almond flour, unsweetened applesauce, vanilla extract, dark chocolate chips, chopped walnuts or pecans, and a pinch of cinnamon if desired.

Stir the mixture until well combined.

Using a cookie scoop or your hands, form small dough balls and place them on the prepared baking sheet.

Flatten the dough balls slightly with the back of a fork.

Bake the cookies in the preheated oven for about 12-15 minutes or until they are lightly golden.

Let the cookies cool on the baking sheet for a few minutes before transferring them to a wire rack to cool completely.

Baked Apples with Cinnamon and Almonds:

What You Need

4 apples (such as Granny Smith or Honeycrisp), cored and halved

2 tablespoons melted coconut oil or butter

1 tablespoon maple syrup (or honey for a non-vegan option)

1 teaspoon ground cinnamon

1/4 cup chopped almonds

How To Make

Preheat the oven to 375°F (190°C).

In a bowl, mix melted coconut oil or butter, maple syrup, and ground cinnamon.

Place the halved apples on a baking sheet lined with parchment paper.

Brush the apples with the cinnamon mixture, ensuring they are well coated.

Sprinkle chopped almonds on top of each apple.

Bake the apples in the preheated oven for about 20-25 minutes or until they are tender.

Serve the baked apples warm, optionally with a scoop of vanilla ice cream or a dollop of Greek yogurt.

Chia Seed Chocolate Pudding:

What You Need

1/4 cup chia seeds

1 1/2 cups unsweetened almond milk (or any non-dairy milk)

2 tablespoons unsweetened cocoa powder

2 tablespoons maple syrup (or honey for a non-vegan option)

1 teaspoon vanilla extract

Fresh raspberries or strawberries for topping

How To Make

In a mixing bowl, whisk together chia seeds, almond milk, unsweetened cocoa powder, maple syrup, and vanilla extract.

Stir the mixture thoroughly until the chia seeds and cocoa powder are well incorporated.

Cover the bowl and refrigerate for at least 4 hours or overnight to allow the chia seeds to absorb the liquid and form a pudding-like consistency.

Before serving, give the chia seed chocolate pudding a good stir to break up any clumps.

Serve the pudding in individual cups or jars and top with fresh raspberries or strawberries.

Berry Chia Seed Pudding:

What You Need

1/4 cup chia seeds

1 cup unsweetened almond milk (or any non-dairy milk)

1 tablespoon maple syrup (or honey for a non-vegan option)

1 teaspoon vanilla extract

Fresh mixed berries (such as strawberries, blueberries, and raspberries) for topping

How To Make

In a mixing bowl, combine chia seeds, almond milk, maple syrup, and vanilla extract.

Stir the mixture thoroughly until the chia seeds are well coated.

Cover the bowl and refrigerate for at least 4 hours or overnight to allow the chia seeds to absorb the liquid and form a pudding-like consistency.

Before serving, give the chia seed pudding a good stir to break up any clumps.

Serve the chia seed pudding in individual cups or jars and top with fresh mixed berries.

Grilled Pineapple with Honey and Mint:

What You Need

1 ripe pineapple, peeled, cored, and sliced into rings

2 tablespoons honey

Fresh mint leaves for garnish

How To Make

Preheat the grill to medium-high heat.

Grill the pineapple rings for about 2-3 minutes on each side, or until they have grill marks and are slightly caramelized.

Drizzle honey over the grilled pineapple rings.

Garnish with fresh mint leaves before serving.

Enjoy the Grilled Pineapple with Honey and Mint as a refreshing and naturally sweet dessert.

Lemon Poppy Seed Muffins (using whole grain flour):

What You Need

2 cups whole grain flour (such as whole wheat or spelt flour)

1/2 cup coconut sugar (or any other natural sweetener of choice)

1 tablespoon poppy seeds

1 teaspoon baking powder

1/2 teaspoon baking soda

Pinch of salt

1 cup unsweetened almond milk (or any non-dairy milk)

1/3 cup coconut oil or melted butter

Juice and zest of 1 lemon

1 teaspoon vanilla extract

How To Make

Preheat the oven to 375°F (190°C) and line a muffin tin with paper liners.

In a mixing bowl, whisk together whole grain flour, coconut sugar, poppy seeds, baking powder, baking soda, and a pinch of salt.

In a separate bowl, mix unsweetened almond milk, melted coconut oil or butter, lemon juice, lemon zest, and vanilla extract.

Pour the wet What You Need into the dry What You Need and stir until just combined. Be careful not to overmix the batter.

Divide the batter evenly among the muffin cups.

Bake the muffins in the preheated oven for about 18-20 minutes or until a toothpick inserted into the center comes out clean.

Let the muffins cool in the muffin tin for a few minutes before transferring them to a wire rack to cool completely.

Mixed Berry Sorbet (using frozen berries and honey):

What You Need

2 cups frozen mixed berries (such as strawberries, blueberries, and raspberries)

1 tablespoon honey (or any other natural sweetener of choice)

1 tablespoon lemon juice

Fresh mint leaves for garnish (optional)

How To Make

In a blender or food processor, combine frozen mixed berries, honey, and lemon juice.

Blend the mixture until smooth and creamy, scraping down the sides of the blender as needed.

Taste the sorbet and adjust sweetness if needed by adding more honey.

Transfer the sorbet to a container and freeze for at least 1-2 hours to firm up.

Serve the Mixed Berry Sorbet in individual bowls or glasses.

Garnish with fresh mint leaves if desired.

Almond Flour Chocolate Chip Cookies:

What You Need

2 cups almond flour

1/4 cup coconut oil or butter, melted

1/4 cup maple syrup (or honey for a non-vegan option)

1 teaspoon vanilla extract

1/4 teaspoon baking soda

Pinch of salt

1/2 cup dark chocolate chips (or dairy-free chocolate chips for a vegan option)

How To Make

Preheat the oven to 350°F (175°C) and line a baking sheet with parchment paper.

In a mixing bowl, combine almond flour, melted coconut oil or butter, maple syrup, vanilla extract, baking soda, and a pinch of salt.

Stir the mixture until well combined.

Fold in the dark chocolate chips.

Using a cookie scoop or your hands, form small dough balls and place them on the prepared baking sheet.

Flatten the dough balls slightly with the back of a fork.

Bake the cookies in the preheated oven for about 10-12 minutes or until the edges are golden brown.

Let the cookies cool on the baking sheet for a few minutes before transferring them to a wire rack to cool completely.

Dark Chocolate Avocado Mousse:

What You Need

2 ripe avocados

1/4 cup unsweetened cocoa powder

1/4 cup maple syrup (or honey for a non-vegan option)

1 teaspoon vanilla extract

Pinch of salt

Fresh berries or chopped nuts for garnish

How To Make

In a blender or food processor, combine avocados, cocoa powder, maple syrup, vanilla extract, and a pinch of salt.

Blend the mixture until smooth and creamy.

Taste and adjust sweetness if needed by adding more maple syrup or honey.

Divide the avocado mousse into serving dishes or glasses.

Chill the mousse in the refrigerator for at least 30 minutes before serving.

Garnish with fresh berries or chopped nuts before serving.

Coconut Milk Rice Pudding with Mango:

What You Need

1 cup jasmine rice (or any long-grain rice)

2 cups coconut milk (full-fat for a creamier pudding)

2 cups water

1/4 cup maple syrup (or honey for a non-vegan option)

1 teaspoon vanilla extract

1 ripe mango, diced

Unsweetened shredded coconut for garnish

How To Make

In a medium saucepan, combine rice, coconut milk, and water.

Bring the mixture to a boil over medium-high heat, then reduce heat to low and cover the saucepan with a lid.

Simmer the rice, stirring occasionally, for about 15-20 minutes or until the rice is cooked and most of the liquid is absorbed.

Stir in maple syrup and vanilla extract.

Remove the rice pudding from heat and let it cool for a few minutes.

Serve the coconut milk rice pudding warm or chilled, topped with diced mango and a sprinkle of unsweetened shredded coconut.

Pumpkin Spice Energy Bites (using pumpkin puree and rolled oats):

What You Need

1 cup rolled oats (use gluten-free oats if needed)

1/2 cup pumpkin puree (canned or homemade)

1/4 cup almond butter or any nut butter of choice

1/4 cup honey (or any other natural sweetener of choice)

1 teaspoon pumpkin pie spice (or a mix of cinnamon, nutmeg, and cloves)

Pinch of salt

Shredded coconut or ground cinnamon for rolling (optional)

How To Make

In a mixing bowl, combine rolled oats, pumpkin puree, almond butter, honey, pumpkin pie spice, and a pinch of salt.

Stir the mixture until well combined.

Roll the mixture into bite-sized balls using your hands.

Optionally, roll the energy bites in shredded coconut or ground cinnamon for extra flavor and texture.

Place the energy bites on a baking sheet lined with parchment paper.

Refrigerate the energy bites for at least 30 minutes to firm up.

Store the Pumpkin Spice Energy Bites in an airtight container in the refrigerator for a quick and healthy dessert or snack.

Baked Pears with Walnuts and Honey:

What You Need

4 ripe pears, halved and cored

1/4 cup chopped walnuts

2 tablespoons honey

Ground cinnamon for sprinkling

How To Make

Preheat the oven to 375°F (190°C) and line a baking sheet with parchment paper.

Place the pear halves on the baking sheet, cut side up.

Sprinkle chopped walnuts over each pear half.

Drizzle honey over the pears and walnuts.

Lightly sprinkle ground cinnamon over the pears for added flavor.

Bake the pears in the preheated oven for about 20-25 minutes or until they are tender and slightly caramelized.

Serve the Baked Pears with Walnuts and Honey warm as a comforting and nutritious dessert.

Chocolate Peanut Butter Protein Balls (using natural peanut butter and protein powder):

What You Need

1 cup natural peanut butter (no added sugars or oils)

1/4 cup honey (or any other natural sweetener of choice)

1 teaspoon vanilla extract

1/2 cup protein powder (use plant-based protein powder for a vegan option)

1/4 cup unsweetened cocoa powder

Pinch of salt

Unsweetened shredded coconut or crushed peanuts for rolling (optional)

How To Make

In a mixing bowl, combine natural peanut butter, honey, and vanilla extract.

Stir in protein powder, unsweetened cocoa powder, and a pinch of salt until the mixture forms a thick dough.

If the dough is too sticky, refrigerate it for about 15 minutes to make it easier to handle.

Roll the dough into bite-sized balls using your hands.

Optionally, roll the protein balls in unsweetened shredded coconut or crushed peanuts for added texture.

Place the protein balls on a baking sheet lined with parchment paper.

Refrigerate the Chocolate Peanut Butter Protein Balls for at least 30 minutes to firm up.

Store the protein balls in an airtight container in the refrigerator for a quick and protein-packed dessert or snack.

Mango Coconut Chia Popsicles:

What You Need

1 cup ripe mango chunks (fresh or frozen)

1 cup unsweetened coconut milk

1 tablespoon honey (or any other natural sweetener of choice)

2 tablespoons chia seeds

Popsicle molds and sticks

How To Make

In a blender or food processor, combine ripe mango chunks, unsweetened coconut milk, and honey.

Blend the mixture until smooth and creamy.

Stir in chia seeds and let the mixture sit for about 5-10 minutes to allow the chia seeds to thicken.

Pour the mango coconut chia mixture into popsicle molds.

Insert popsicle sticks into each mold.

Freeze the popsicles for at least 4-6 hours or until they are completely frozen.

To remove the popsicles from the molds, briefly run the molds under warm water to loosen them.

Serve the Mango Coconut Chia Popsicles as a refreshing and tropical dessert on a hot day.

Chapter 5: Final Thought

As we conclude our culinary exploration of the world of endometriosis, we find ourselves at a juncture where sustenance, empowerment, and a deep understanding of the role of food as a potent ally in navigating the challenges of this condition converge. This cookbook endeavors to offer a holistic perspective on the intricate connection between food and health, transcending mere consumption to encompass nourishment of the body, mind, and spirit.

The recipes, reflections, and insights contained within these pages serve as invaluable resources that have the potential to enhance your well-being and elevate your quality of life. Crafted with care and consideration, the recipes featured herein are crafted to provide not only physical nourishment but also emotional solace and support as you chart your individual path towards managing endometriosis.

Armed with the knowledge gleaned from the Endometriosis Diet, may you be empowered to make informed decisions that promote hormonal balance, alleviate inflammation, and alleviate pain. It is our sincerest hope that these recipes serve as catalysts for both physical and emotional healing, reminding you that food has the power to infuse joy and vitality into your life.

Furthermore, remember that you are not alone on this journey. A community of individuals who share similar experiences, seek answers, and believe in the transformative potential of food stands beside you. Your resilience and determination thus far are a testament to your strength and tenacity in embracing each moment, even in the face of adversity.

I am deeply grateful for the opportunity to share this cookbook with you as you embark on your journey. May these dishes not only bring you pleasure and nourishment but also ignite a renewed sense of vitality and resilience as you experiment and create in the kitchen. With each meal, may you find comfort in knowing that you are nurturing your body, soothing your soul, and harnessing the healing power of food.

As you continue your journey with endometriosis, may you find solace in the knowledge that you are supported, uplifted, and empowered by the nourishing embrace of food every step of the way.